Level Up

A Guide to Cleansing the Mind, Body, and Soul

Benevolent Blizz

Editor: Sharp Editorial, LLC

Cover Image: @VegThug on Instagram

Please Be Advised

The content in this book is designed to provide helpful information regarding various health topics. This book is not meant to be used, nor should it be used, to diagnose or treat any medical condition. The advice in this book is strictly for educational purposes and personal research only. The author, editor, and publisher are not responsible for any health or allergy needs that may require medical supervision, and they are not liable for any damages or negative consequences from any action, application, preparation, or procedure to anyone reading or following the information in this book. References are provided for informational purposes only.

Table of Contents

Dedication

This is dedicated to everyone who took the time to read this book to better their lives.

I would also like to dedicate this book to my beautiful queen and princesses. Also to my amazing editor, Laci, with Sharp Editorial. Without them, I could not have made this book possible!

Introduction

One summer afternoon, in 1998, when I was just 15 years old, I was able to score a ride home from what was my first ever (and last) summer school experience. I piled into a Subaru Outback, along with five other friends. I called "shotgun," a term calling "dibs," on the prime front-passenger seat, but another one of the passengers said he already had dibs on it. I wasn't too happy to give it up, but I was happy to have a ride, nonetheless. So, behind the driver I went with three of us in the back seat and one in the hatchback. The next thing I knew, I woke up on the curb, bleeding from my face, with my shoes off. I was not quite sure what happened. We made it less than a mile from summer school before the driver lost control of the vehicle, fishtailed, and flipped into oncoming traffic. Two of the passengers in the car were killed, and the driver of the truck involved was killed as well. A mother and her two children were also struck, but they were not seriously injured. The passenger next to me died in the crash as well as the rider in the shotgun seat that I had attempted to claim. The story of this accident made the front page of *The*

Washington Post, and every local news station came to my home to ask for an interview.

I was a mischievous and troubled youth, yet always very smart with a great deal of common sense. I was kicked out of many high schools and wanted nothing more than to play basketball. I was only in summer school so that I could go back to school during the regular year and play basketball. However, my pelvis was fractured after the accident which led to me being on crutches, not able to walk much, and definitely not able to dunk a basketball. I had previously been able to dunk a basketball at the age of thirteen. All of these changes sent me into a downward spiral.

At fifteen years old, I had been involved in a deadly accident, and I was required to stay in the hospital for a short stint before being released. When I was finally released, I was sent home with my "dime bags" of wacky tobaccy (cannabis) that I placed in my underwear before the accident. After the accident, the hospital staff had cut off all of my clothing, placed me on a gurney, and eventually received an x-ray of my pelvic region. My pelvic region is where the wacky tobaccy was, and it was amazing to me that I was released with the same bag of cannabis that I had on me before we crashed. I always wished that I could thank all of the paramedics and doctors who chose to turn a blind eye to that, especially given all of the media coverage.

Having two of my classmates pass away in the same car that I was in really hit home, and I knew I was spared for a reason.

The thought that I was spared for a reason never went away but, honestly, it took me a while to fully appreciate or take meaningful action in my life to make good on it. Sometimes, I lost sight of the fact that "I was here for a reason." Fast forward to ten years later, I still had cannabis on me, and I was heavily drinking and sleeping until 2 pm, every day. Fast forward a few more years, at 31 years old, when I had my first child. Her birth led me to research vaccines for her two-month-old pediatric visit. This opened the door for me to research all things relating to food as nutrition and corruption. By the time my daughter was six months old and moving to solid foods, she and I started a vegan lifestyle.

The day I stopped eating animals, life started to change rapidly for the better. I still did not quite understand my purpose, but I knew I was on track.

Several years later, present day, I have written three books and most certainly found my purpose. The point of this introduction is to give you honest insight into my previous life and self and how I got to where I am now by fulfilling a dream of helping others live a healthy and happy plant-based life. What changed my life was becoming conscious of all things that I intake via my plate and subconscious and conscious self. This book will help you learn how to combine the two, causing you to level up your life and the lives of those around you.

Namaste,
Benevolent Blizz

Preface

"I healed my disease, pain, anger, and depression with more bacon," says no one, ever!

That statement *has* been repeatedly said. However, you must replace "more bacon" with "a holistic lifestyle."

I have healed my dis-ease, pain, anger, and depression with a holistic lifestyle, and many others have, too. Many have never looked back after they transitioned; after all, they are too busy ascending.

Once upon a time, I was a stereotypical American on a typical American diet, which led to standard American results – dis-ease, pain, anger, and depression. After all, I was consuming unhealthy, processed foods and drinks, so I was hardly surprised at what became of my diet and lifestyle. I did not have a technical disease diagnosis. In retrospect, however, I was a ticking time bomb, on edge, sluggish, frequent headaches, back pain, and unhappy; thus, dis-eased. Now, on a plant-based diet, I avoid the word "bomb," as it is destructive and having to do with war. Plant-based, holistic living is all about choosing life. So, life I speak, write, and think!

Glossary

<u>Break-fast</u>: a term used to intentionally show that breakfast is breaking your nightly fasting period

<u>Dis-ease</u>: a term designed to intentionally remind you that disease is the body not at a state of ease

<u>Hueman/Huewoman</u>: a term used to remind you that we are all one man and woman under the sun, just different shades and hues of skin color

<u>INI</u>: a term used to describe and encapsulate both you and me as one in the same; similar to a reflection

<u>Inner-G</u>: a term used to describe one's inner strength, energy, knowing, and determination

<u>Innerstanding</u>: having a firm grasp on information or knowledge, not under or beneath you as in understanding

<u>Ital</u>: natural

<u>Livet</u>: a term designated to differentiate itself from a standard American diet (SAD – one based on consuming dead things) to a plant-based livet (based on living foods and life)

<u>Mylk</u>: a term used to describe plant-based milk, setting itself apart from traditional animal milk

Level Up

Namaste, my good people!

This manual will share all I have learned and have been blessed to download into my mainframe which, in turn, improved my life ten-fold and propelled me to ascend to a higher level of consciousness and wellness. We all experience different situations and circumstances in life which contribute to our level of awareness. Regardless of where that level may lay right now, there is room to level up and ascend.

With that said, I have compiled the steps that took me from being a self-centered, stagnated, depressed being to a person who will not allow a negative thought to take up my mental. I share the inner workings of a person centered on service to others, exhibiting ideas of service with blessings flowing abundantly while staying mindful of emotions, only choosing thoughts that beneficially serve my life.

The information provided can help anyone, at any level of consciousness, reach their highest potential. In an easily understood and applied manner, I will teach the power of understanding your mind, body, and soul as well as how to apply the Law of Attraction to live holistically. You will learn how to ascend to your fullest, healthiest, and holistic life through the power of your life (body), the power of your thoughts (mind), and the power of the divine and unseen (soul).

What one should know is that this ascension is easily attainable because this is already in you (inner-g) and is something everyone is born with in their souls. I am simply here to help you tap back into your divine self.

I will start by addressing the food that goes into your body and placed on your plate because you are what you eat. If you eat sick, depressed, sad, angry, or fearful energy via food, you will develop one or all of the characteristics above. It's a new day and age, and you must adapt if you want to thrive. Thus, you must start with what is on your plate.

Food is the most important factor of this elevation process, and I will give you a pertinent example as to why. I know many enlightened and spiritual individuals who do not have the desired health or body that they wish. One cannot simply meditate or do yoga to achieve holistic health. You can do as much yoga and meditation as you please, but if you continue to ingest poison, you can become and remain diseased. Just the same, you can eat as much kale as you please but if your thoughts are not at ease, your body will be diseased. You can do crunches until you develop a ten pack, however, if you are not considerate of your livet and mind, you will become and remain diseased. The point is, you need to incorporate a holistic approach for optimal health. Thoughts, prayer, and meditation are extremely powerful, but they cannot work instantaneous magic to the point of turning poison to nutrients. This is part of the reason you must first examine your plate and diet and change it to a livet. It's akin to putting an oxygen mask over oneself first, thus being able to help others. Healthy food and a clear gut will free the mind. Changing what is on your plate will open many doors and awakenings for you. Once again, you have to put the mask over your face, first, before you can help anyone else; you cannot help friends, family, or animals if you are not in proper health. So, start with the plate.

Please keep one important thought in mind before I continue to discuss plate, diet, livet, and the effects on the mind – energy is constantly in motion and never ceases to rest. Thus, energy cannot be destroyed, only transferred. Think about what that really means and what type of energy the meat in your refrigerator carries. If the animal is killed and slaughtered, it will carry energy of fear, anger, depression, and destruction. Remember, energy can only be transferred, not destroyed, so this is where "you are what you eat" comes into play. The energy from the vibrations of fear, depression, and anxiety from your consumed animal products must become you as there is no escaping this upon ingestion. Add synthetic growth hormones, antibiotics, arsenic, carbon monoxide, and other carcinogens, and now we are talking about a ticking time bomb dumped into your body which is heading down the path of disease and destruction. This is why ingesting foods with a high vibration is vital. There is a type of photography, Kirlian photography, which measures the energy emitted from various items or, lack thereof, like cooked food and meat. Cooked foods emit a considerably lower vibrational aura compared to raw fruits and vegetables, which literally radiate life force energy. A piece of cooked meat has little to no life force emitting from its image. This is because heat changes and destroys the life force energy of matter, especially raw (living) food. Enzymes are key, and enzymes are destroyed when heat is put to food. Raw foods are loaded with enzymes and nutrients that one should leave intact, raw at all costs. When you flood your body with enzymes and phytonutrients, you repair at a cellular level. Cooking food negates much of this power. Cooked vegetables also emit a much lower vibration than that of their raw counterparts. You must keep in mind that food grown on the green Earth is already cooked to perfection by the sun. This is known as sun-fired foods. I credit the term "sun-fired foods" to the man who coined the term and is recognized as the grandfather of gourmet raw cuisine, Aris Latham. I have also learned the idea behind break-fast that I will later share in this book as well as several other aspects of my nutritional knowledge that I learned from Aris Latham. I have learned much from Aris Latham, but what stuck out the most, and this is what I teach most often, is that you must wash your insides (internal) as much or more than you wash your external (ass/behind). He worded this advice more eloquently, but wording it like this has already stuck in the minds of many others. "Wash your insides as well as you wash your ass." With that said, I will now examine the body – how to detoxify it, how to build it, and how to naturally and organically blast off when connecting the mind and encompassing in the soul.

Namaste.

Body

Morning/Break-fast

When considering the body, you must keep one important thought in mind, and that is you are being bombarded with an array of toxins on a daily basis. Keeping this in mind, and having a good innerstanding of the toxins you are exposed to, will help keep you conscious of what goes in the temple.

You are exposed, daily, to an assortment of chemicals, from the air you breathe to the water you bathe with to the water you drink.

The air and water you breathe and drink truly put a new meaning to fresh air and water. Geoengineering, more commonly referred to as chemtrails, is now a conspiracy reality that can no longer be denied and swept under the rug. Chemtrails and air are two factors you have no control over; you can choose water and food but not air. As if looking at the sky was not enough confirmation, the government has now admitted to stratospheric injections which they claim is for climate control and global warming. For example, there have been soil samples that draw parallels with government-planned means of injection of barium, strontium, aluminium, and other chemicals in a chemical cocktail to replicate that of a volcanic ash which cools the atmosphere. Many soil test samples, in what used to be some of the most untouched areas like Mount Shasta, show large and unusual amounts of heavy metals such as strontium, barium, and aluminum. Combine that with air pollution from factory farming, factories, and car pollution, and now we are talking about a new meaning to fresh air. I am not one to fear monger and introduce a problem without a solution, so here are some quick, heavy metal chelation tips.

Heavy Metal Chelation

There are different ways to go about heavy metal chelation or detox. Some of the best ways are by juicing with an abundance of parsley, dill, and cilantro, especially, which is proven to attract heavy metals from the body like a magnet. Another highly effective tool is chlorella powder. When buying chlorella, you may want to avoid buying chlorella from China, as it could be contaminated from the Fukushima radiation fallout. Yes, Fukushima happened in Japan, but effects from the fallout have been seen as far as

California, and a large percentage of chlorella comes from China. You can also use herbs, such as burdock, made into a tea. Additionally, you can use other herbs such as milk thistle, dandelion leaf, moringa, and chaga mushroom. Bentonite clay and activated charcoal can be used to detoxify the body as well. Another powerful tool is intermittent fasting. Intermittent fasting is when you allow the body an extended period of rest from processing and digesting food, allowing the body time to detoxify.

Water has also been compromised. Besides your breath, what is more important than the food, air, and water you consume? Of course, little to nothing comes close to importance in comparison to air, food, and water. This is why it is vital to develop a firm innerstanding that all three resources have been compromised so that you may have the greatest level of awareness moving forward. Tap water is full of hundreds of chemicals, but there are three highly detrimental chemicals.

Out of the hundreds of chemicals in tap water, three of the most toxic are lead, atrazine, and fluoride. Lead contamination is not a problem isolated to Flint, Michigan. Basically, every major city has high concentrations of lead, with water fountains as the common culprit. This is because, like many water infrastructural systems and pipes, they eventually become corroded or outdated. I am from Maryland, just outside of the nation's capital, Washington, D.C. I was born and raised in D.C., so I am well aware of the track record of D.C. tap water, and a quick, funny story will tell the tale of how long this has truly been a problem.

I remember a time in elementary school, around the fourth grade, when I was mixing a large glass of powdered Lipton ice tea with a large glass of D.C. tap water. I chugged it, and two minutes later, the headline on the nightly news was "Boil. Tap Water is Tainted." So, this has been a problem as long as I have been alive. Lead, like barium, strontium, and aluminum, is a neurotoxin which accumulates in the brain and is highly detrimental to brain development in children.

A scientist from The University of California, Berkeley was hired by the company that produces atrazine to study the chemical compound (Hayes, 2010). His results were shocking. When male frogs were exposed to atrazine, they turned to hermaphrodites, displayed homosexual tendencies, and repelled from female counterparts, thus unable to reproduce. Other hormone disruptants, such as

BPA and soy, which are forms of synthetic estrogen, are found in almost everything via soy byproducts and plastic.

The last of the three major detrimental chemicals is fluoride. Fluoride, which many are unaware, is another neurotoxin. Many are under the false impression that fluoride is not only beneficial but necessary, and this, much like almost everything else we are told, could not be further from the truth. Remember, it is always Opposite Day in Babylon. If something is beneficial, it is banned by the Fraud and Deception Administration, also known as the FDA, while poisonous neurotoxins are added to the drinking water in mass quantities. So, what exactly is fluoride, anyway? Have you ever asked yourself or do you have any clue? Fluoride is a byproduct of the phosphorus mining industry.

- Several states classify fluoride as hazardous waste.
- Fluoride is the only unregulated drug that is forced as a mass medicine on people with no control of dosing or frequency, supposedly to prevent tooth decay (Zelko, 2018).
- In 2012, Harvard researchers listed fluoride as one of the top developmental neurotoxins on Earth (Choi, 2012).

- Twenty-seven studies showed a connection between fairly moderate exposure and lowered IQ in children (Choi, 2012).
- If ¼ mg of toothpaste is ingested, you are advised to call Poison Control. The same amount of fluoride is in one cup of tap water.
- Forty-one percent of children have fluorosis, which is excess fluoride on the teeth, resulting in white patches and discoloration, also affecting neurotransmitters (98% of EU opted not to fluoridate water) (Beltran-Aguilar, 2010).
- Big business – fluoride is sold back as a byproduct to chemical treatment facilities.
- Teach your children not to swallow.

There is no logical reason to mass medicate the water for the sake of cavities. Do you really think the government cares that much about your teeth? You have two of the most damaging neurotoxins known to man in your drinking water. Do you really think that there is not a numbing and dumbing down of the population? Heavy accumulation of an array of heavy metals as neurotoxins could cause one not to be able to think critically and make proper connections. It's all by design that you are in a brain fog and unable to piece the matrix codes together. It's critical that you understand you are being attacked at all angles, by the water, air, and food, so that you will truly understand the importance of living a detoxifying lifestyle, not just a random detox, as this does not address the problems.

Food

Let's briefly touch on how your food supply has been hijacked. This subject is vast, and I will elaborate in the "Genetically Modified Organisms (GMOs)" section, but for now, here are major examples of how your food supply has been bought out where profits trump health and integrity.

First, let's discuss the soil that our food is grown in which is a major problem. The soil has been depleted through the heavy use of pesticides and synthetic fertilizers. Soil test samples show unusually high levels of heavy metals. The cause and effect is that produce is now shown to have a depleted vitamin and mineral content. So, our fruits and veggies are now nutritionally void, which is a problem, even if you are adding lots of these to your diet or livet. To compound the problem of nutritionally-void produce, this produce is further deteriorated by cooking all of the life force energy out of the food. Not only is the food depleted to begin with, and many people are not eating as much veggies as they should in the first place, but it is generally further depleted by the cooking process. Again, keep in mind that heat destroys enzymes and nutrients.

This is where our slow speed masticating juicer becomes so critical to help us supplement the void!

We live in a country where most of our food is banned in the majority of other countries. Instead of a ban of genetically modified foods, we live in a country where the opposite happens, and corporations lobbied and succeeded in passing laws *not* to label GMO foods. Instead of banning them, it's always Opposite Day in Babylon. By banning the labeling of GMOs, the Fraud and Deception Administration thought that consumers should not have the right to know if they are consuming GMO foods.

Take French fries, for instance. One would think French fries contain potatoes, salt, and oil, and if you were in Europe, that would be correct, but in the heart of Babylon (U.S.), there are 17 ingredients in McDonald's fries, many of which you can't pronounce and some of which are known carcinogens. This is just in the "potato" French fries, so imagine what's in the burgers. You've got to love the good ol' Fraud and Deception Administration that bans cancer-healing treatments such as cannabis oil and Vitamin B17 while allowing doctors to treat cancer with another poisonous method proven to have a 5% success rate (chemotherapy). The United States is a place where your meat is grown with antibiotics and growth hormones. Then, after being slaughtered, the meat is treated with carbon monoxide to avoid the rotting carcass turning brown and then subsidized to ensure the "meat" is affordable enough to keep the beast system going. Wouldn't subsidizing fruits and veggies make more sense?

Did you know that nearly all antibiotics in the U.S. are used for factory-farmed animals? Did you know that some chemically-treated meats can be shipped to China for processing and shipped back to the United States without labeling its origin? Look into Codex Alimentarius, a set of guidelines of nutritional standards resulting in the nutritional dumbing down of the entire food supply from supplemental dosages to ineffective levels to irradiating all food products to no longer have truly raw foods.

Once upon a time, organic food was referred to as food. They use words to mislead consumers into believing that foods sprayed with toxic pesticides are conventional and those grown naturally deserve a special name and higher price tag. Keep in mind, all ingredients found on shelves and in fast food places are first deemed safe by the FDA. Ingredients such as artificial colors, dyes, GMO ingredients, and MSG, all hidden in thousands of different ways, are deemed safe. This should help you realize that the FDA does not have your best interests at heart, and you must take your health into your own hands. Otherwise, you will be led astray. Remember, FDA = Fraud and Deception Administration.

With building up a better understanding of the on-going deception and daily ingestion of toxins, let's discuss how to live a detoxifying lifestyle, getting back to that amazing and life-changing concept of washing your insides as well you do your ass. This starts in the morning with your break-fast or lack thereof.

Benevolent Blizz Intermittent Juice Fasting Protocol; Body-Morning/Intermittent Fasting

This is the most important part of your livet and detoxifying lifestyle, and this is the key to weight loss. Intermittent Fasting (IF) is also the key to keeping weight off and the key to major daily detoxifying and regeneration, which should be part of your morning routine.

The most important part of the day is break-fast, but like most of the time in Babylon, this is a half-truth. Break-fast is the most important part of the day, but not in the way this half-truth is portrayed. If you do not eat a monster breakfast, would you wither away? No, quite the opposite.

Many are intimidated by the concept of fasting. After all, we live in a gluttonous society, and if you were to go on a fast, you would certainly die of protein deficiency and wither away, right?

Wrong.

Let's explore this fasting concept for a moment. To begin, do you realize you go on a fast, every day during your sleep, without consciously realizing it? That fast ends the moment you put food into your mouth at break-fast. Well, this meal, first thing in the morning, also stops your body's repair and regeneration process. The moment you put food into your mouth, the repair process has stopped, and the vital organs and intestines go back to work. The key to major detoxification, cellular and DNA repair, regeneration, and weight loss maintenance is your morning routine and intermittent fasting (IF). IF allows your body to continue the repair and regeneration process.

Think about the times you felt sick. Your body automatically tells itself not to eat so the body can heal. Overeating is the number one problem that gets in the way of healing. People heal by going on juice fasts, giving the body a chance to heal instead of working on constantly digesting foods. Adapting IF into your daily lifestyle will truly change your life. So, how do you go about having an internal shower while intermittent fasting? The answer is simple: juice fasting, every morning, which will technically turn IF to I juice F. This is how you expedite the regeneration and healing process while flooding the body and cells with an abundance of nutrients – a win-win with multiple benefits.

You can go about internal showering and scrubbing in a few different ways. Upon rising, drink as much water as you can possibly consume. To give a certain ounce amount is silly because we are all different sizes, and long-hand math is also unnecessary. Simply put, drink as much water as you possibly can upon rising. You can add lemon, lime, or sub-acid fruit. These ingredients will have an alkalizing effect on your body. Normally, you would stay away from any fiber to extend the fast. Fruit in water, or the form of pulp in fruit or melon juice, is the only exception to including fiber during intermittent juice fasting. Fiber from fruit acts as an astringent while veggie fiber is high in cellulose and a bit more difficult for the body to break down. Fruit fiber will also speed up bowel movements. When consuming heavy liquids while IF/juice fasting, you will urinate often. This is a sign that you are filtering properly. You also are releasing toxins.

So, begin with as much water as you can possibly consume. Wait 15 to 30 minutes, and move on to a green or fruit juice. A sample morning could look like this:

- 8:00 am – Drink as much water as you can
- 8:30 am–9:00 am – Chaga
- 9:30 am– 10:00 am – Fruit/melon juice (fruits digest fastest next to water, so it is best to consume fruits before green juice)
- 10:00 am – Green juice

This timeline is interchangeable but best executed in the order mentioned above. You can drink more or fewer ounces of juice in the morning and then enjoy break-fast around noon with water-rich fruits, chia seed cereal, or gluten-free oatmeal.

So, as you can see, IF/daily juice fasting is not difficult. You are basically extending your daily sleep fast for a few hours after waking and stopping any solid food from going into your body after 8:00 pm. This gives you an eight-to-ten-hour window of intake and building, but more importantly, a 14-to-16-hour window of rest and repair.

One to two days a week, I will make juice for three days. If you do not have juice made on a given day, you can switch it up with water and herbs. Juicer types are later discussed in the "Juicers" section.

Once you understand your circadian rhythm cycles, and understand break-fast is a period of elimination, you will realize this process is actually very normal.

Now, let's explore the opposite, more typical, sad diet-morning routine. Within thirty minutes to one hour, food has crossed the mouth, stopping the repair process before the elimination process has finished or taken place. The morning is time for elimination via bowel movements and urination. Mid-day and afternoon should be your main building period, and winding down occurs in the evening, not eating heavily, having your meal close to bedtime when your body goes back into the rest and relaxation period. Your body works on three, eight-hour cycles referred to as your body's biological clock or circadian rhythm. 4 am to noon is your body's elimination period via pee, poop, and sweat. Noon to 8 pm is your body's building period. This is the time in which you can come in with as many pure, plant-based whole foods as you would like. 8 pm to 4 am is your body's rest and rejuvenation period. Your body works on elimination, build, and rest cycles. These cycles are based upon the sun and moon, day and night. Thus, there is no cheating the circadian rhythm. There is only cheating thyself. For example, those who work the "graveyard" shift have higher rates of mortality. Going against your circadian rhythm will also set you up for a pattern of gluttony by expanding your stomach.

There is a night-and-day difference between these two routines. One promotes weight gain and to steadily add taxing work on the body's temple (and intestines), and the other routine is exactly the opposite because it promotes weight loss and keeps the body lean and shredded while flooding the body with nutrients that cleanse and detoxify the intestines. IF does not constantly tax the body because this routine does not involve ingesting foods such as bacon, egg, and cheese. IF gives the temple and intestines a much-needed break to handle more important tasks such as regeneration. Now you can better understand the power and importance of juice and IF. There are many different styles, methods, and levels of IF, and I suggest figuring out what works for you and your schedule. Remember to flood the body with fresh water, juices, and herbs, for as long as you can, and do not sweat the clock or math. Specific details of juices and herbs to consume in the morning are discussed later in the book; for now, let's move on to the topic of solids.

Break-Fast Solids

At this point, if you have followed the guidance above, you have already taken an internal shower and washed your insides better than your ass. Now you can move on to understanding the power of solids. There are a number of health-conscious, plant-based options to consider for your solid breakfast such as fruit, smoothies, oatmeal, pancakes, and so on. My favorite, and the most nutritionally dense choice, is chia seed cereal, also known as chia seed porridge. This is a blend of chia seeds, hemp seeds, and flax seeds along with fruit and homemade nut mylk which covers all the bases and is loaded with bio-available protein and healthy omega-3s. It also tastes great and is child-approved.

Thus far, you have given your body an internal shower and flooded your cells with an abundance of vitamins, minerals, chlorophyll, and nutrients; you've had heavy elimination, and you moved on to intake bio-available and healthy fat-packed foods with fiber, and it's only noon! At this point, going down this livet route, you have already served your temple better than most will the entire day.

Let's review the difference in a sad diet breakfast. A sad breakfast likely consists of the following:

- Processed animal products (categorized by the World Health Organization as a class-one carcinogen)
- Starch and gluten (acting as glue in the body as it does in bread)
- Eggs (one of the highest sources of saturated fat and cholesterol)
- Cheese (ultra-processed and pasteurized dairy)
- And maybe a glass of hormone puss and blood in the form of cow milk.

Step back, think, and ask yourself why you are eating this and where on Earth is the nutrition? When eating a sad breakfast, how much fearful, negative energy have you taken in before noon?

Anyone who knows anything about fasting knows it makes no sense, scientifically, to break a fast with heavy, fatty, solid foods. Your body should always *ease* into breaking your fast, and that should be done with liquids, building up digestive enzymes, prior to indulging and building.

Now, take the time to compare a sad breakfast to that of a plant-based livet with a juice break-fast. The decision should become much easier and clearer. Hopefully, you will choose life.

At this point, you can indulge in as many plant-based, high-vibrational foods, as this is now the building cycle of your circadian rhythm. Building foods such as quinoa, chickpeas, nut butters, avocados, and plenty of vegetables, leafy greens, and sprouts are high-vibrational foods that will raise the body's vibration. Remember, you are what you eat.

You may be wondering what to do with these glorious foods. For more detailed recipes, please stay tuned for my *7-Day Recipe Book*. This book will provide mid-day and dinner meal ideas to help you structure the better part of your day.

You have vast options to choose from in the plant-based kingdom. As mentioned above, there are foods such as quinoa, which can be utilized in many different ways. Simply boil water, add quinoa, turn the heat down, and simmer until the water evaporates. You can add anything from sautéed kale and maple-glazed sweet potatoes to black beans and bell peppers to BBQ jackfruit. The options are endless, and this is just for one combo. A combo with a quinoa base makes anything you add a proper food combination. Quinoa is a complete protein in itself. In short, starch is digested starting in the mouth, and protein is digested starting in the stomach which can cause a traffic jam in your belly resulting in gas, bloating, and irritable bowel syndrome (IBS). For now, let's move on to more mid-day meal suggestions.

Becoming gluten-free is not only a response to sensitivity or disease, nor is becoming gluten-free only for hippies and soccer moms in South Beach. Gluten-free is not a fad! To an extent, we are all gluten insensitive as we are all lactose intolerant. However, we have different levels of sensitivity. Nevertheless, let me be clear – gluten should not be consumed in the human body, and gluten should be avoided the same way one may avoid drinking the milk from another species like a cow. Gluten acts like glue in the body, the same as it does in breads and pastries. Gluten is essentially a binder, and it acts as such in the body. Gluten bogs the body down the same as pasta bogs the body down; pasta equals paste.

Gluten = glue

Pasta = paste

I have a saying that goes: *gluten is glue; it bounces off of me and sticks to you* (your love handles and gut!)

Many people who had no apparent signs of gluten sensitivity, after becoming gluten-free, noticed it was difficult to go back to consuming gluten once they have been given the opportunity to feel the difference.

Another detrimental aspect of gluten is that nearly all gluten is derived from wheat and has been riddled with known carcinogens from pesticides and herbicides such as roundup glyphosate. GMO's will be further discussed in the "Genetically Modified Organisms (GMOs)" section.

Now that you have a better understanding of why you should avoid gluten, let's discuss gluten-free options.

For just about every food, and I mean every food, there is a gluten-free version.

You can find yummy, gluten-free bread like millet and flax bread or chia seed-based bread. You can use gluten-free almond flour tortillas, coconut wraps, and veggie wraps, or you could make a scrumptious raw, vegan, gluten-free onion bread. With the options above, you have many bases to use in place of gluten. You can make a PB&J with gluten-free bread and kick up the nutritional value by swapping peanut butter for raw cashew, almond, walnut, or coconut butter. You can up the nutritional value, again, by using fresh fruit for jelly. I enjoy using raspberries and blackberries and mashing these berries with a fork. Bam! That is our jelly or jam. Top your sandwich with hemp seeds, and you will have a tasty, nutritious sandwich. This is child-friendly, too. You can also use this same recipe in a coconut wrap and swap the berries with bananas and dates. Also, you can eat this at any time of day. There are so many gluten-free ideas such as grilled cheese, tempeh or hempeh sandwiches, chickpea wraps, spread sandwiches, avocado toast, hummus, and jackfruit sandwiches. The options are endless.

You can create similar meals with gluten-free almond flour tortillas, such as black bean quesadillas, cheese quesadillas, and any plant-based variation you could imagine. Keep in mind, with any packaged product, read the ingredients. When it comes to vegan cheeses, all are certainly not equal. You will get what you pay for; the cleaner, of course, the better. Many dairy-free cheeses are full of ingredients that certainly do not serve your temple. Vegan cheeses are often nut- and seed-based cheeses, and these cheeses, along with herbs and spices, should be the only ingredients. Avoid cheaper brands with ingredients like canola oil, modified starches, and natural flavors.

You can create many meals with lentils such as high-vibrational soups, stews, or Sloppy Joes. You can also make curry chickpea stews and chickpea spreads. Once again, there are many directions one could go. However, your best option is a pure salad, and not your average, run-of-the-mill, bland iceberg lettuce and shaved carrot rabbit salad with toxic dressing on top. I'm referring to kale, spinach, or a 50/50 spring mix as the base. There are many ingredients to add such as heirloom tomatoes, which is one of the healthiest foods on Earth; purple onions, which are very powerful, antiviral, and anti-bacterial; pumpkin seeds, which are anti-parasitic; sunflower seeds, which are a good source of protein; and strawberries and dates which are good sources of minerals and iron. Plus, they sweeten a salad. You can also add raw soaked nuts such as Brazil nuts or cashews which are a good source of healthy fats and protein. You can add paprika and adobe for flavor. For salad dressing, I opt for homemade, as most store-bought dressings are full of additives and preservatives. You can make a quick and easy dressing by simply mixing equal parts of raw, unfiltered apple cider vinegar, avocado, or hemp oil, plus mustard and maple syrup. Whisk together with a fork, pour over salad, massage, and thoroughly mix all ingredients with love.

For dinner, the sky is the limit, yet again. Anything you used to eat with dead animal products in it can easily be veganized. You will want to check out my upcoming cookbook for recipes such as gluten-free butternut squash lasagna with almond ricotta, smoked mozzarella stuffed chickpea patties, curry chickpea stews, homemade pizza, empanadas, eggplant parmesan, shepherd's pie, and spaghetti squash with homemade nutballs. Whichever route you go for your dinner meals, keep it plant-based, highly raw, and vibrant as possible, only using cooking oils like avocado and sesame and being aware of different smoke points of oils, many of which should not be cooked with like coconut oil and hemp oil. These oils have low smoke points, after which they become rancid. At the point they become rancid, free radicals are formed, and free radicals are like thugs to your cells! Coconut, extra virgin olive oil, and hemp are all amazing, beneficial oils that must be consumed raw.

As long as one has a well-rounded, whole food, plant-based livet, iron deficiencies and inflammation should not be a problem. I would, however, suggest taking a Vitamin D and B12 supplement because Vitamin D is what truly keeps you thriving, especially in the winter when there is a lack of sun. B12 ensures proper brain and nerve function. Keep in mind – there is no such thing as cold and flu season in places where the sun is abundant. Also remember to keep your food gluten-free, not overcooking and destroying veggies, avoid processed foods and processed refined sugars, and eat no later than 8 pm and no sooner than two hours before sleep. Then, you will find yourself in optimum health.

Food as Medicine

The basis of holistic health, physically speaking, is that food is your medicine. Ensuring that the vast majority of what you eat is high vibrational, preferably organic, pesticide-free, and whole alkaline foods will keep the doctor away.

If you feel the need to visit a doctor for whatever ailment or reason, consider that you know your body best; for non-life threatening events such as a minor cold or other ailments, consider being your own doctor. The food and beast system is purposely designed to keep you a customer for life to Mr. Big Pharma. Antibiotics are overused so much that super bugs are becoming prevalent, and these bugs are becoming increasingly resistant to man-made, synthetic drugs. You must keep one very important fact in mind – the body is organic and extremely displeased when attempting to metabolize anything synthetic.

Alkaline Acid

Your body is constantly working to maintain a proper pH balance. In chemistry, pH stands for potential hydrogen. The pH scale ranges from zero to 14 with zero being the lowest level of acidity. Fourteen is the highest level of alkalinity. Your body is constantly working to remain in an alkaline state. When you move to the acidic side of the scale, you move to the dis-ease state. Acid foods promote mucus and inflammation. Alkaline foods promote detox and rejuvenation, and also make it very, very difficult for any dis-ease to live in temple! This is why it is a must to consume a highly-alkaline livet.

Powerful Herbal Supplements

Bioavailability is key, and ital is vital. I have three powerful tools to get you through a cold, flu, bugs, and viruses without building up any tolerance. Three go-to herbal remedies have served my family and me well. These three methods are extremely powerful, safe, effective, and multi-purposeful. They are fire cider, elderberry syrup, and oil of oregano.

Fire cider is apple cider vinegar on steroids. It is a fermented elixir with an ACV base with a mix of peppers, horseradish, ginger, turmeric, onion, garlic, and raw honey. Note: Raw honey is the only non-vegan product I will consume because benefits outweigh the negatives. With that said, the only time I would consume honey would be as medicine in the fire cider or elderberry, not as a common sweetener.

Fire cider is a rather potent combination that works in synergy to combat any cold or flu. It is also a fermented beverage, so it has benefits for the stomach as well as adding pita (fire) to the stomach which basically gets the digestive system primed and ready. Also, fire cider is great for the respiratory system and safe for children, as long as you can convince them to swallow.

Elderberry is proven to kill a cold and the flu as well. Elderberry syrup is a great cough suppressant for children as well as adults. Elderberry is a supreme immune booster and has a pleasant taste for children. You can buy syrup from your health food store, and you can purchase elderberries from the local herb shop. Make these into a tea or boil down to make your own syrup.

Oil of oregano (OOO) is basically anti-everything. OOO is antibacterial, antiparasitic, and antiviral. It kills eczema, psoriasis, and toe and nail fungus, and it boosts the immune system. Oil of oregano basically kills everything. Viruses and bacteria are like little creatures that try to invade, rob, and take advantage of the temple while the OOO is like the OG that steps in and puts them back in check. OOO may be used as a bug repellent when diluted and mixed with a carrier agent like avocado or coconut oil. Five to ten drops of OOO to two to three tablespoons of carrier oil works well as a bug repellent.

OOO is also great for killing parasites and candida, which may be wreaking havoc on many people. To remedy this, consider going on an oil of oregano regimen for six months, one month on and one month off, and see how you feel. To do so, take four to eight drops, internally and incrementally, working up to a full dropper at a time for one month. Then, assess. I'm sure you will notice many improvements. When the parasites exit your body, you regain control of your body and cravings, and you also gain clarity, as the parasites control the gut which is correlated to brain function.

Consider this – when buying OOO, buy one standardized to 70% carvacrol or p73. If going on a regimen, consider a probiotic to assure proper gut balance and flora as the oil of oregano does not discriminate in killing and, over time with extended use, can also kill some good bacteria. This is why taking off every other month is suggested. This should not worry or scare you away, as it is extremely safe, and when one is on well-rounded, organic, high-vibrational, whole foods, plant-based livet, there should be little to no concerns.

Supplements

The only supplements I recommend are Vitamin D and Vitamin B12. Again, when on a well-rounded, high-vibrational livet, supplements are not needed. Green juice is the best multivitamin one could ever take. You must remember that the body cannot metabolize synthetic pills and supplements; most are a waste of money and literally peed down the drain. There is no such thing as cold and flu season, but there is such thing as lack of Vitamin D, otherwise known as lack of sunshine and lack of nutrition. You will notice that there is no such thing as cold and flu season in the tropics, Caribbean, and warm climate environments. The abundance of sunshine is key.

Regarding the Vitamin D supplement, keep in mind that if it is not a vegan Vitamin D3, then it is more than likely from lanolin (sheep's wool). *Yuck.* Imagine that picture for a moment – fresh wrung sheep's wool. You want to look for a clean source of vegan Vitamin D. Dosage depends on the amount of sun, or lack thereof, but due to geoengineering, the sun is commonly blocked out in most parts of the world regardless of temps. So, for adults, aim for 2-5000 IU, daily, from fall to the beginning of spring; for children, aim for 1000-1500 IU, daily. When sunshine becomes more abundant in your area, you can scale back to 2000 IU per day for adults, and 1000iu for children.

For your Vitamin B12 supplement, the key is to find methylcobalamin, not cyanocobalamin. Cyanocobalamin requires the body to convert B12 back into methylcobalamin. Much of the vitamin is lost during this conversion process. Aim for around 2-3000 mcg, daily. Good, plant-based sources include chlorella and vitamineral green. Chlorella and vitamineral green are the only other supplements I would consider, but not necessary. Chlorella is one of the oldest living organisms which has not changed form in millions of years. Chlorella is a good source of chlorophyll and protein and a great heavy-metal detoxifier.

Herbs

When researching herbs, understand they are for healing. Next to juicing and fasting, herbs are the king of all healing tools. There are so many herbs to choose from to heal just about any ailment or disease. I recommend researching or searching the ailment and herbs to "help." A sample search may be "herbs to help with inflammation" or "herbs to boost iron." A wonderful fact about herbs is that they are extremely safe, and mostly affect children in the same, safe manner. Herbs are also very effective. Explore my "Herbal Remedy Handbook" (set for release in 2019) for a specific breakdown of a broad spectrum of herbs.

Below is a list of some of my favorite and most used herbs, but I also encourage you to reference my "Herbal Remedy Handbook" or research the vast herbal kingdom.

- Burdock for iron and blood cleansing
- Valerian/catnip/lavender as a sleep aid
- Dandelion as a digestive aid and multivitamin
- Nettle for your multivitamin and pregnant women
- Moringa for energy and as a multivitamin
- Elderberry and elderflower for an immune booster, cold and flu, and cough and congestion
- Lemon balm, holy basil, and red rose for calming and relaxation
- Ashwagandha to balance hormones and stress
- Marshmallow root powder and slippery elm are both good for digestive assistance, throat-coating, and repairing a leaky gut
- Chaga for adaptogen; it contains one of the highest antioxidant level of any source on Earth and the highest source of melanin

- Solomon seal for adaptogen, inflammation, and joint recovery
- Maca for energy, vigor, and vitality
- Horsetail for shiny, strong, and healthy hair.

One quick side note on the cannabis herb, which has many medicinal and therapeutic benefits – your chosen method of consumption matters. When you put fire to the cannabis plant, all medicinal value is lost; actually, the opposite happens, and carcinogens are released. This comes from the fire turning flower to ash, therein lies the carcinogens. Additionally, when the herb is commercially grown, it is grown for profit, thus likely grown with an abundance of synthetic pesticides and fungicides, often resulting in an abundance of undetectable mold. To compound the issue, the herb is often placed inside tobacco cigars which are known carcinogens. Opt for unbleached organic papers. Using a vaporizer, such as a volcano vaporizer, drastically reduces carcinogens, too. If you want to level up from there, consuming cannabis via a clean, vegan edible is the next most health-conscious way to indulge. Topical salves also work well for inflammation and joints as well as CBD.

The next step in enjoying the true medicinal value in cannabis is in juicing the fresh bud leaves which has no psychoactive effect.

Lastly, the ultimate medicinal value is in the cannabis oil, otherwise known as Rick Simpson Oil, full-extract cannabis oil (Feco), or Phoenix Tears. Although the FDA has not approved these statements, there are many testimonials available from people reversing multiple, varying dis-eases through a cannabis oil regimen.

Fish (to Eat or Not to Eat?)

Long answer in short, no. There are many issues with the current state of our oceans and fish supply.

Farm-Raised Fish

Unless advertised differently, most of today's fish consumed in restaurants and fast food chains are farm-raised. There are many problems with farm-raised fish. To start, their diet consists mostly of GMO corn and grain which is not only extremely unnatural but also void of nutrients. Salmon are dyed pink, as they are originally an unappealing grey color. Studies link farm-raised tilapia to negative effects on the heart from saturated fat levels compared to that of bacon. Also, similar to the chickens and cows, farm-raised fish are fed antibiotics and growth hormones, as they are often bred in unpleasant, man-made farm ponds in countries thousands of miles away with lax regulations and standards over the farming operation.

Wild-Caught Fish

I often hear people claim only to eat wild-caught fish. Somehow, these people missed the memo that wild-caught fish is also detrimental to thy temple.

Their home in the ocean is highly contaminated to start, thus making the fish highly contaminated. The oceans have become a dumping ground from heavy pollution, chemical waste, oil spills, and radiation fallout, and the fish are unable to avoid contamination. Also, many of the fish sold and consumed are bottom feeders, ingesting a lot of matter that you would never want to ingest. Wild-caught fish are not only full of worms and parasites but also full of mercury. Keep in mind – as I write this, in 2018, Fukushima is still leaking radioactive material into the Pacific Ocean. So, take extra caution to avoid fish from the Pacific Ocean. The vast benefits touted in fish, such as omega-3, are not only fully bioavailable from fish but are easily obtainable from a more bioavailable source by cutting out the middleman. When cutting out the middleman, you will flourish more.

Parasites

The discussion of parasites is a good transition from fish which are loaded with parasites. I am frequently asked about parasites. Just about all of us are carrying hosts. These parasites control our urges and appetite. Getting rid of parasites is crucial to clean the gut, which, in turn, will free the mind. Mind, body, and soul – always connected.

These parasites and hosts love to feed on sugar and animal protein. Cutting off their life supply should make a non-conducive environment for them. There are other tools you can use to rid the body of parasites, as mentioned before, such as going on an OOO cleanse or regimen every other month for six months or so. Take four to eight drops of OOO, every day, working up to a whole dropper full at a time. Other great tools to rid the body of parasites are pumpkin seeds and papaya seeds.

Genetically Modified Organisms (GMOs)

GMOs should be highly avoided on a wholistic livet towards ascension. GMOs are genetically modified foods, made by man and not by nature. GMOs have never been studied long-term, and studies that have been conducted result in large and abnormal tumors in lab rats and mice. GMOs are banned in many countries. On the other hand, labeling is banned, so consumers are uninformed and not deterred from GMO processed foods.

Most GMO foods are built with a pesticide roundup in the seed. This same roundup, when ingested by the pest, causes the pest's intestine to explode. This pesticide is linked to many cancer studies. Many countries have banned the selling and cultivation of GMOs. However, one of the most telling signs of GMO displeasure and unacceptance to those that know better may be the story of Haiti and GMO seeds. Haiti, one of the world's poorest nations, refused and burned Monsanto GMO seeds.

Say "no" to GMOs.

Go organic, and if you want to upgrade from there, go to your local organic farmers' market. From there, the ultimate standard is that of growing your own food.

Endocrine Hormone and Disruptants

There are several hormone disruptants in today's food and water. Let's talk about a few of the most common. Hormone disruptors throw hormones off balance and wreak havoc on your endocrine system, causing all sorts of problems such as mood swings, sexual impotence, low sperm count, and many other bodily issues.

Some of the most common endocrine disruptors are BPA, atrazine, soy, and mercury. We already discussed atrazine in detail in the "Water is Life" section and, assumedly, most know the dangers of mercury, which is in the top five most toxic substances on Earth; so, let's focus on BPA and soy.

Soy contains phytoestrogens that mimic estrogen in the body, and the vast majority of soy is genetically modified. To make matters worse, most soy products are heavily processed. If you are going to consume soy, I recommend organic and of a fermented variety like tempeh or miso.

BPA vs. BPA-Free

Bisphenol A (BPA) has chemicals in it which replicate synthetic estrogen. Plastic contains BPA, and when coming in contact with the skin, BPA is then absorbed into the body. The most common culprits of BPA exposure are from plastic via plastic bottles and the lining in canned foods. The BPA is leached from the plastic bottle from temperature fluctuation, heating, and freezing, and leached through can linings from acidic foods like tomatoes which marinate in the BPA. However, there is another common culprit of BPA exposure and that is the form of receipts, specifically gas station receipts. Every time you are handed a receipt, you up your exposure; so, a simple "no thank you" to receipts will drastically cut down on exposure. A 2003-2004 study conducted by the Center for Disease Control showed that up to 91% of Americans have BPA in the body.

BPA-Free Marketing Scam

You may say to yourself that you will be careful with the receipts, and that you are already using a BPA-free water bottle. This marketing ploy once bamboozled me until I dug a bit deeper. BPA stands for Bisphenol A. Companies merely swap one endocrine-disrupting compound, BPA, for another endocrine-disrupting compound in bisphenol-b through Z. This replacement compound is less studied but has already been shown to be as detrimental as BPA. The alternative is to use glass. Choosing glass is a good transition to the best type of drinking water.

Drinking Water

The best drinking water to consume can become a heated debate. First, let me say that the best way to consume your water is to eat it. Eating your liquids through liquid-based fruits and veggies like melons and cucumbers, which are all in the 90% water range, gives you an abundance of vitamins, minerals, and electrolytes with pure AKA distilled water.

Let's talk about distilled water for a moment.

When discussing distilled water, the first thing someone will say to you is that distilled water leaches minerals. These people likely have never looked further into that statement. This, like many concepts in the matrix (Babylon), is a half-truth. Distilled water does leach minerals, but what they conveniently forget to tell you is that distilled water leaches inorganic minerals. Distilled water creates a negative charge as do organic minerals.

Inorganic minerals, on the other hand, have a positive charge, thus attracting to each other like a magnet. Distilled means pure. All water in nature is distilled. Water in fruit is distilled. All vegetation in nature is watered with distilled water. Distilled water is one of the ultimate secret tools of healing and detoxification. Many of the healthiest elders I look to, who look decades younger than their birth age, have been drinking distilled water for decades, people such as Annette Larkins, John Rose, and Aris Latham, to name a few.

Aris Latham, master teacher and raw vegan for over 40 years, looks decades younger than his actual age, and he only drinks coconut water. This is another great source of distilled water which somewhat resembles that of human blood plasma, and it is loaded with one of the highest sources of electrolytes. On a well-rounded livet, minerals should not be needed from your water, and water should not be a go-to source for minerals. Minerals in water are essentially tiny microscopic rocks picked up from the top of the spring. These go into the body as tiny microscopic rocks, much of which are inorganic minerals, thus storing in joints and leading to arthritis. The next best option for water would be reverse osmosis which is the next closest to pure water.

Avoid bottled alkaline waters as they are nothing more than a marketing scam due to the fact that they are always in plastic bottles leading to leaching BPA and acidity; thus, this water is not alkaline. One quick and easy tip to boost the alkalinity effect of water in the body and remineralize water is to add lemon, lime, berries, dates or your fruit of choice. Lemons and limes have an excellent alkaline effect on the body. Fruit also contains vitamins and minerals and adds great taste to the water. If you do not own a distiller, you can refill quality water from your local health food store. Remember to refill in glass!

Juicers

Juicers can vary in price and style, and deciding among them may become a bit overwhelming and confusing; so, I will try to simplify. When considering juicing, the biggest benefit is that you can get an abundance of raw vitamins, minerals and, most importantly, enzymes. The most important factor to consider in juicing is retaining enzymes. When looking for juicers to buy or upgrade to, look for slow-speed-masticating style juicers. Many masticating juicers run at a very slow speed or rotations per minute (RPM). Eighty RPMs would be one of the lowest on the market which means that the slower it's running and rotating, the lower RPMs it generates. This can also turn the shelf life of your juice to three to five days instead of as soon as possible or same day. The lower the RPM, the slower the juicer, and the more potent and higher quality your juice will be.

I do not recommend juicing too many fruits, as this concentrates fructose and discards fiber which further harms the body's regulation and distribution of fructose. This is where the differences between juicing and blending become important.

Juicing vs. Blending

Juicing and blending have distinct benefits. Juicing provides the body with a concentration of nutrients, without any fiber, giving the digestive system a much-needed break from overeating and overindulging while flooding the body with chlorophyll and an abundance of nutrients from fruits and vegetables.

Blending has its own benefits, specifically when it comes to fruit. When dealing with fruit, you do not want to concentrate the fructose and discard fiber. Fiber helps regulate the fructose, therefore stopping the body from going on a roller coaster ride, so to speak, from unregulated fructose. Blending also can be a great way to fit a large amount of protein into one liquid setting. For example, smoothie form. Smoothies can also be used to promote weight gain, which is a good transition to our next topic, gaining weight on a plant-based diet.

Gaining Weight on a Plant-Based Diet

For many people, losing weight and maintaining weight loss is a common goal for going the plant-based route. Obesity has become a common problem in society, so many folks are already going into a plant-based livet, needing and wanting to shed some weight. There are others who already have a thin body type and may want to gain weight, while others may lead an active lifestyle or may be an athlete requiring a higher caloric intake. This is where the blender comes into play, helping you gain weight, as you can pack an abundance of calories and protein in an easily digestible, bio-available way via smoothie. So, let's discuss some of the tools you can use to gain weight.

I would not worry about actively trying to gain weight, as you should appreciate that you do not have the opposite issue, trying to lose weight, which can be much more damaging. Just as society has corrupted self-image, that is no different for that of the skinny body type wishing to appear more macho or tough (masculine) or "thick" for a woman. This is a psychological issue that must be addressed. As long as you are eating a whole-food livet, conscious of foods, thoughts, and exercises, one should not fret.

However, the key to gaining weight is taking in more calories than you are burning. You can monitor this by looking at your activity and energy level and addressing accordingly.

The following are great food choices for healthy weight gain:

- Nuts
- Seeds
- Avocado
- Coconut and cashew butter
- Almond and almond butter
- Walnuts and walnut butter
- Hemp seeds
- Chia seeds
- Pumpkin seeds
- Sunflower seeds
- Bananas
- Fruit
- Chlorella
- Spirulina
- Spinach

- Beans
- Lentils
- Mushrooms
- Chickpeas
- Hummus.

Many of the above mentioned are high caloric foods and/or high in protein. Many of the above mentioned can also be easily added to a blender to form a smoothie. If you are looking to gain some weight, consider intermittent fasting for one hour less per morning.

Circadian Rhythm

Circadian rhythm is akin to the body's internal clock, working on a cycle that tells the body when to eat, sleep, and eliminate. The circadian rhythm can affect weight loss and weight gain, as well as affect your sleep pattern. The body works on three-hour cycles:

- Restoration cycle from 8 pm–4 am
- Elimination cycle from 4 am–noon
- Building cycle from noon–8 pm.

Eating into the elimination cycle or sleep and restoration cycle will lead to weight gain. This is the key to weight loss. Your circadian rhythm also affects your sleep cycle and tells your body that the time has come to go to sleep and wake up. Blue screens such as cell phones, laptops, computers, and televisions negatively affect your sleep cycle, making it harder to fall asleep, keeping you awake longer but also hindering your deep sleep.

Deep sleep is vital for your body to repair and regenerate. Tossing and turning are signs of a lack of deep sleep, thus a lack of proper cellular regeneration. Wi-Fi can also affect deep sleep and circadian rhythm. Before you go to bed, unplug your Wi-Fi modem and try to not stare at screens before bedtime. Getting in tune with your circadian rhythm is vital for peak performance ascension health.

Reading Labels

You will avoid a vast amount of problems by eating the rainbow and eating whole foods that are the ingredient, not containing ingredients, but let's be honest and practical – you will likely purchase packaged foods. When buying products with multiple ingredients, therein lies one of the major keys to avoiding booby traps and chemical shit storms and that is buying products with as little ingredients as possible. More ingredients are likely to be more processed which is likely to increase the chances of GMOs and chemical consumption. So, first thing first – buy the cleanest products available on the market, and remember, the longer the shelf life, the shorter it makes ur life.

Keep in mind that ingredients are listed by weight. The first ingredient is the ingredient most prevalent by weight. Avoid products when oil and sugar are the second, third, and fourth ingredient because this indicates too much oil and sugar for a product, more than likely comprised of 50% sugar and/or oil.

Avoid canola oil, in particular, as this is a man-made oil derived from the GMO rapeseed. Non-GMO canola oil is yet another crafty marketing ploy. It took scientists over ten years to lower the uric acid levels of canola to a somehow acceptable FDA standard that should actually be highly avoided.

Refined sugars should also be avoided. Refined sugar affects the brain similarly to cocaine and is as much or more addictive than cocaine. Other ingredients to avoid include:

- Artificial and natural flavors
- Colors and numbers such as blue 40
- Ingredients with protein at the end such as pea protein
- Modified food starches
- Carrageenan
- Ascorbic acid should also be avoided because this acid commonly derives from black mold.

All of these "ingredients" have multiple health risks like neurotoxins and endocrine disruptors, but what is most common among these ingredients is the fact that most contain multiple proprietary ingredients like natural and artificial flavors, colorings, and protein, and they all contain multiple ingredients in themselves. Avoid them at all costs.

What Goes on Your Body Goes into Your Body

When discussing how to read ingredients, I want to remind you that whatever goes *on* your body goes *in* your body. Many people may look at food ingredients but assume their skin is like a shield instead of what realizing what their skin really is – a sponge. A general rule of thumb is that if you cannot eat a product or put it in your mouth without harm, then you likely should not put it on your body. Over half of the water from a shower is absorbed into the body. To make matters worse, cosmetics and fragrances do not have to list ingredients, and most are comprised of chemicals. One of the most important items to avoid is deodorant because it is full of aluminum and parabens.

Your armpits are one of your only ways to execute elimination. Your body wants to expel toxins, not trap them in with another toxin in aluminum. Another bit to consider would be using chemical-free and fluoride-free toothpaste, chemical-free hand and body soap, and chemical-free laundry detergent. When you wash your clothes with carcinogenic detergents, thus toxin is transferred to clothes, thus transferred to the skin, thus transferred into the body. Also, one should be mindful of inhaling toxins via air fresheners, plug-ins, and so forth. If you can smell it, you are ingesting these artificially-scented items.

DIY Considerations

Nature always has the answers. Nature always knows, and nature always nurtures, and these very simple and effective DIY products made from natural ingredients are examples of nature's remedies. The more one detoxes and becomes less and less toxic, items like deodorant will not be needed or needed less frequently. You can make your own deodorant by simply rubbing half a lime on your armpits. You can make your own toothpaste with baking soda, coconut oil, and essential oil. You can make your own disinfectant in a spray bottle with lemon, lime, apple cider vinegar, and water. You make your own bug repellant with a couple of drops of oil of oregano (OOO) per tablespoon of coconut or avocado oil. For anything else in between, I recommend Dr. Bronner's products and Meyers products for your body, dishware, and clothing. Remember, avoid aluminum parabens and fragrances!

Body in Summary

You can summarize the body ascension part of the trifecta easily. Don't over think it. Eat at as many organic, high-vibrational whole foods as you wish within your circadian rhythm. Avoid chemicals and processed foods. Consider intermittent fasting or a period of time for a solid food vacation. Wherever you are at this point, whether consuming dead animals, consuming transitional plant-based foods, or an on-and-off healthy eater, strive to level up, aiming for whole raw foods as the brunt of your livet.

Use food as medicine; thus, any disease from hypochondria to whatever the case may be healed via one's plate in conjunction with one's thoughts, both of which will be discussed in the "Mind" portion of the book.

Namaste.

Mind

One cannot begin to be health conscious without what first?

A thought.

Everything begins with a thought.

Thoughts are so powerful that they can cause or cure disease, as shown by the placebo effect when unknowing recipients of tests are fed sugar pill instead of said medicine and cured by the power of their thoughts alone. Negative thoughts produce a substance in your body called cortisol. Too much cortisol production will cause dis-eases to manifest in the body. This is why you can eat as much alkaline food as you want until your hair turns green, but if your thoughts are not positive, your physical body will not be healthy either.

Connecting the Dots

This section is where you start to piece together the mind and body connection. You cannot have complete health without a full mind-body connection. Let's take a look at a couple of examples of why the mind, body, and soul connection is so important for overall physical health.

Let's say you want to vibrate higher, you want to ascend, and you want peak performance health, so you are eating all the alkaline foods in the world until your hair turns green yet you are not waking up to do a meditation to set your tone for the day to mitigate stress. This absence, in turn, could raise cortisol which would negatively affect your overall health. Now, let's say you are eating all the alkaline foods in the world, trying to vibrate higher and reach the healthiest version of self, but you do not do a two-minute stretch upon rising. You may experience stiffness, which may lead to back pain, which will lead to poor health. Let's say you are attempting to develop your physical with weight training. You are doing crunches until you have abs, but you are not combating stress through positive thoughts and watching your plate. Well, you could become dis-eased and perish with that same build and abs. You cannot have complete health without the complete trifecta. You cannot obtain true health just from the plate, as you cannot obtain true health just from thought, as you cannot obtain true health just with meditation or exercise, just as you cannot fully ascend and vibrate higher without the thoughts to match the wanted vibrations accomplished through meditation. You must understand, you cannot have complete health without the complete trifecta.

When you take a step back and become more aware and conscious of your mind and thoughts, you may discover they can be downright ugly. People often carry many negative thoughts about others and themselves. Many of these negative thoughts and beliefs have been inside for so long, and people are not aware of them anymore yet they are living off of their subconscious reaction.

Controlling Emotions and Taking Power Back

You must try and be mindful of the fact that only you have the power to make yourself angry. The power of your thoughts and emotions is one thing no one can or should be able to take from you. When you let someone make you angry, you have lost control of yourself, essentially becoming a puppet on a string. Ask yourself – do you ever really want to be angry? Of course not. You give that power to someone else because if it were left up to you, you would not allow yourself to feel such unpleasant emotions that you can control. It's never the person, place, or situation but your reaction to the person, place, or situation. Take control of your emotions, and take full control of your life.

There is always a blessing and learning experience in any and every negative situation. Through the hard times, adversity, and life experiences, you are handed learning experiences, and when you are handed the learning experiences, you can upgrade and progress. You would not experience growth if not for the failures and bumps in the road. The secret to surviving and thriving is in living and learning from the experiences, thus comes wisdom. There is little use for knowledge, only a seed planted. Without applying the knowledge in the planted seed, information is not useful.

Applied knowledge = wisdom.

This is where you learn to tap into the power of your mind and the Law of Attraction (LOA) to magnetically attract what you want by tuning into the same energy frequency of what you desire. Think of your cellf as a radio. You can't tune into rock and roll on the frequency of classical, can you? So, you cannot expect to tune into the frequency of appreciation and positivity on the frequency of complaining and negativity. Thoughts become reality, so if you focus on the negative, sickness, anxiety, and fear, those feelings will become you. Change the way you look at things, and the things you look at start to change!

Thoughts are things, and thoughts shape your reality. Everyone's reality is based on their current level of perception, which could also be called your level of awareness. This is why ignorance is not bliss, especially when it comes to natural law. Natural law sheds no grace for ignorance. You either are aware and able to work with the universe or you are not aware and will thus violate the law at every turn. You can only do as well as what you are aware of. The less aware you are, the more ignorant one will be. Perception is key. This topic circles back to shaping your reality and being able to take the good from a seemingly bad situation, all by changing your perception. One must master the art of transmutation, turning all seemingly bad to positive. Realizing that all seemingly bad situations are learning experiences will help master the art of transmutation.

Mind-Like Computer

The mind is like a computer processor. It only has so much room for so many gigabytes, and most of our memory storage is filled up with television, social media, news, work, and other day-to-day tasks. This is why it is hard for one to receive new downloads, because the mind is filled with the anti-social media, friends, entertainment, music, and so forth. It is important to be mindful of what goes into your brain, otherwise known as your Pentium processor. Think about how long you have been letting these outside sources program your Pentium processor. You must take back control of your thoughts and mainframe. I will say this ten times over in the "Mind" section alone – your thoughts equal your reality. You are not only what you eat but also what you think. If you think you can't do something, you cannot. Simply change the belief, and now you can move that much closer to your goal. This is how your conscious and subconscious work together, by repetition and scrubbing the old junk. All you have to do is be willing to change your beliefs and change your life. Change the way you think, and you will change your life.

Conscious and Subconscious

The subconscious knows no difference between good, bad, right, wrong, rich, poor, negative, or positive. The subconscious accepts whatever you tell it. The subconscious does not know the difference between a penny and a million dollars. It accepts whatever you tell it. You are living off of your subconscious, 99% of the time, based on reactions. Positive conscious thoughts are overrun by much larger subconscious programming. This is why it is so important to scrub the subconscious, delete all outdated programming, Trojan horses, and bugs, and consciously reprogram with positive affirmations. So, how do you go about cleaning, erasing, and reprogramming?

Scrubbing – Subconscious Protocol for Reprogramming

This section is very important because we step into the process of change. The power of positive thoughts will not work if your subconscious programming does not match. This is also why it is critical to scrub the old programming from your subconscious. The brain is like a tuning fork. If I send out negative vibes, it will not resonate with anything good. There is no such thing as coincidence; what I send out, I get back. Choose wisely.

There are different tools you can use to scrub your subconscious. First and foremost, you must be conscious of what goes into your mainframe, just the same as you are conscious of what goes into your body via plate. You must be mindful of what you listen to and watch such as the news, music, radio, and so forth. These outlets shift your programming, thus shaping your life.

The law of energy states that everything is moving and nothing is at rest. If you were to look at your body under a microscope, you would see cells moving. You must match your vibration and energy with that of what you want to attract. You must tune into your body.

Affirmations

Affirmations are one of the greatest tools you can use to scrub and tune the subconscious. The problem, once again, is the negative programming you have been told and lied about and even told and lied to yourself. How many times have you told yourself the following:

I could never do this!

This will never work!

I'm too stupid!

I can't do this!

Needless to say, these affirmations have a negative effect on your programming.

Imagine repeating positive affirmations, over and over:

I am able.

I am making this work.

I am enough.

I am smart.

I am healthy.

I am attracting major success, prosperity, abundance, and peace into my life.

This positive programming is the idea and basis behind affirmations. You are reprogramming the subconscious and conscious to the new, positive programming by repetition. Just as you repeatedly told yourself negative, self-limiting thoughts and ideas, you must repeatedly feed yourself new programming. Reprogramming will not take a lifetime of scrubbing and undoing, but it will take some time. Through affirmations and meditation, which I will discuss more in depth, in conjunction with stopping the intake of detrimental programs for your mainframe, one can blastoff and flip tables at a rapid pace.

The Power of "I Am" and Letting Go

The power of "I am" and affirmations are likely the greatest tools you have to scrub the subconscious and conscious. Every cell responds to every thought you think and speak. The body is a mirror of your beliefs. Continuous modes of thinking and speaking produce body behaviors and eases or dis-eases. There are problems you can solve and those you cannot. So, there is no need to worry about a problem you cannot solve, and just the same as it is useless to worry about a problem you can solve. This is, again, why keeping positive thoughts is so important. A lifetime of negative programming will take some time to reprogram. You can reprogram, daily, just like you detox, daily, by using affirmations and "I am." Replace phrases like "I can't" or "I will" with "I am." You will find a considerably faster route for reprogramming by replacing "I will" with "I am." If you have not physically started towards your goal, "I am" will manifest sooner than the "I will," which often never comes. If you hold the "I will" or, worse, the "I will one day," you will be stuck in "i willville" purgatory as the universe will match what you constantly declare, "i will one day". So, I will one day, forever stuck in one day. The same goes for focusing on the lack thereof in your life. If you focus on the lack thereof, you will create more lack thereof. Where the focus goes, the innergy (energy) flows.

There is a huge gap between "I will" and said goal. Simply moving to "I am" visualizes you that much closer to said goal. "I am" is a command and declaration to the universe.

There are people to help you with the power of affirmations, if need be, such as Louise Hay. Louise Hay has easily been one of the most influential teachers in my life, and when it comes to the power of thought, she has been the most influential. Her greatest lesson was the gift of forgiving and letting go. This is a gift to oneself, first and foremost. When you forgive and let go, you free yourself. Often, the person you are angry with or hold resentment towards may not even know. They may be in control of your emotions, and neither party was ever conscious of it. Imagine that. Forgive, let go, and free thyself. Reprogramming without releasing old blockages is extremely hard. To release old blockages, you must address history and trauma.

Forgiveness is a gift to yourself. When you forgive and let go, you are free. Again, the person you are angry with or resentful toward may not know, yet that person may be in control of your emotions and not conscious of it. Forgive, let go, and free thyself.

Addressing the Old

You cannot move forward and ascend while holding on to old baggage of hurt, anger, and resentment. You must bring this darkness to the light to cleanse and transmute it. Again, you must address to progress, and you must amend to ascend! One wanting to ascend must master the art of transmutation. Transmutation is turning negatives to positives in all areas, all ways, and always!

One of the best ways to address the old and, more importantly, in a safe and controlled, non-volatile setting is by doing so during meditation. Once again, this allows you to keep a safe setting that does not have to become confrontational.

Forgiveness Exercise

Do a meditation, and draw the top three people to your mind that you have unresolved resentment towards. Tell them you love them and you are sorry, regardless if you feel you are in the wrong or the one that needs to apologize. Then, forgive this person, without the need for punishment; this is true forgiveness. Lastly, let go.

There is an abundance of resources available on YouTube for guided meditation. Visualizing old hurt and trauma may stir up emotions during meditation and may lead to tears. This a great sign that you have addressed old baggage and released some blockage, but not to fret if no tears have been shed. Stay the course, and repeat the affirmations, over and over again. Use powerful affirmations such as the following:

I am enough.

I am willing to change.

I am healing.

I am healthy.

I am happy.

I am appreciative.

Remember, when addressing old trauma, releasing blockages, forgiving, and letting go are gifts to yourself. Keeping this in mind to forgive and let go.

Hooponopono

The Hooponopono prayer is another powerful tool you can use to forgive and let go. Hooponopono is an ancient Hawaiian prayer that is simple yet powerful:

I'm sorry.

Please forgive me.

Thank you.

I love you.

This is not only an extremely powerful forgiveness tool, but Hooponopono is also an extremely powerful concentration and visualization technique. You can apply the Hooponopono to any aspect of life, not just for others but to forgive yourself. Use the Hooponopono to forgive yourself for any situations or instances you hold against thyself, times you continue to hold yourself guilty, times you may have used money or food to oppress others, times you used your wits for unrighteous gain, and times you caused someone else to be in a negative situation to better your life. Forgive yourself as much as you work on forgiving others.

Resentment

When you do not forgive and let go, you form resentment, and resentment is one of the most destructive emotions you can carry. Moments of anger can sometimes last for short periods of time yet still be highly destructive. Now, imagine the destruction of resentment, essentially a constant form of anger, and how that negatively affects your body. Resentment literally eats at the body. Resentment increases cortisol levels which cause dis-ease. Avoiding this is a major benefit of letting go. Is a grudge worth your physical health?

Appreciation

Once you innerstand the power of thoughts, realizing that you must address old issues to move forward, you must write the reprogramming. The reprogramming starts with your thoughts, words, and appreciation. The new programming must start with love, appreciation, and gratitude, as love is the highest vibration and the answer to all, and appreciation is a life hack to bring you more. These two feelings, next to the plate, are the most powerful tools for ascension. Love, appreciation, and what you eat are the trifecta for triumph. The power of thought and appreciation are also the combination for success with the law of attraction or the law of magnetism.

Universal Law/Law of Attraction

The world is run by universal laws where there is never any cheating, and there is no bypassing. They are in place, 24/7, on the east, west, north, and south, day and night, and universal law is not manmade so there is no changing or cheating universal law! Universal law sheds no grace on your ignorance. You either know and work in accordance with the law and win or you violate the law at every turn by being unaware of the law. Knowing this is a big step to living righteously. Once one is aware of natural laws, knowing there is no escaping or cheating this, it is impossible to do wrong to others. Knowing this is a big step to living righteously, knowing that you have essentially done something to yourself and it is sure to come back via the law of karma and the LOA. Having a firm grasp on universal law will help you immensely in all areas of life. The world is run by these laws, first and foremost. First thing first is morals. Nothing else matters without morals. All universal laws can be summed up, in short, by doing no harm to others, living righteously, and doing what is right, period. We all know right from wrong. The LOA, in particular, has more intricacies to be able to apply successfully.

LOA – Words are Swords

To apply the LOA principles, properly and effectively, it is helpful to have a firm innerstanding on the power of words. You now understand the power of thoughts, and words are just as powerful as your thoughts; they go hand in hand. It's vital to have a good innerstanding of how energy and vibrations work. You must be in vibrational alignment with that of what you desire. Imagine your body, once again, and that you are a tuning fork. You want to tune into the station of abundance, prosperity, success, and happiness, but your vibrational frequency (radio station) is tuned into that of complaining, negativity, anger, and what you are lacking. The only thing you can attract is that which you are in the vibrational frequency of. So, the universe matches your vibration and gives you more anger, negativity, and lack thereof! Where the focus goes, the energy (inner-g) flows. So, tie the power of thoughts and words together to change your body's radio station (vibrational frequency). This is also where faith starts to intertwine with the body and mind.

Remember, everything begins with a thought. Thus, this is how you change your vibration. What you put out you get back. The concept is summed up that straightforwardly. As above, so below, as within, so without, the vibration inside of you will match what you outwardly attract.

Another good tool to use is imagination – imagine and speak as if whatever you want has already occurred. For example, I am building a multi-million dollar empire. I have multi-million dollar ideas which lead to other multi-million dollar ideas. I am attracting more abundance into my life.

Now, one must stay the course to change one's frequency. This is not a magic trick. This practice does not work like that. You must keep the subconscious scrubbing and hold the manifestation to be already true. Each thought starts as a weak vibration. With enough time and focus, those weak thoughts become dominant thoughts, and dominate thoughts become manifestations!

The rest is easy; stay righteous, stay the course, and stay in the highest vibration which is love and appreciation.

At this point comes the truly beautiful part because you can now sit back, enjoy the ride, and let life take over, knowing life and the universe always has your back and is in full support of your dreams. That only occurs when you live by the law, the natural universal law.

It will be extremely helpful if you keep in mind, while tuning into your desired frequency, that words are swords and spelling cast spells. There is no spelling without the word spell. This, alone, should remind you how powerful your words are and to choose wisely.

Masuru Emoto conducted amazing experiments with the power of words, energy, intent, and their effects on water. Dr. Emoto found that water that was spoken to with love formed perfect geometric crystals when froze, and those water samples spoken to negatively formed odd, uneven patterns. Now, keep in mind that your body is largely comprised of water. So, how are you speaking to your body?

He also found that the water exposed to classical music formed perfect geometrical patterns. In contrast, that of heavy metal music produces similar results to tap water in not being able to form solid geometric patterns. This shows the power of words, thoughts, intentions, and energy.

Words are energy.

Words are a form of magic.

Magic has a strong relation with magnetic and electrical energy. Take "net" out of magnetic and see that you are left with magic. Take "ing" off of spelling and you are left with spell. Take the "s" off of swords and you have words. This is no mistake. Words are swords.

Master Teachers

While I have a very firm grasp on the mind, energy, and the LOA, it would be a disservice not to mention and acknowledge the master teachers I have learned from. The person whom I learned the most about the power of thoughts is Louise Hay. Louise is considered by many to be a modern-day saint. She occupies a wealth of knowledge, but what I learned most from her is to forgive and let go. Forgiveness is a gift to yourself that frees you; from there, you can reprogram and hold the vibration of love. She taught me that you must heal yourself first. Then, you can apply the law of attraction to your life.

Other influences such as Napoleon Hill, Bob Proctor, Wayne Dyer and Abraham Hicks are master teachers of the power of thought and the LOA. Once you begin to align your plate and power of thoughts, life will automatically change and new worlds will open for you. Change the way you look at things, and the things you look at will start to change. From here, you will begin making connections, bring the sight unseen to light, and start to trust the sight yet still unseen.

Soul, Spirit, Sight Unseen, and Now Seen

Once you transition to a high-vibrational livet and align your thoughts with your high-vibrational livet, the universe takes over, and it is likely that your level of faith in the universe will guide you to the sight unseen. Things you cannot physically touch like your spirit, your soul, instinct, your third eye, your intuition, your (ancestral) and spirit, and angel guide may manifest in number and numerology which is a good start to tap into the soul.

Numerology (1111, 33, 44)

Numerology is a great way to tap into the soul, the divine, your guides, and the sight unseen. I receive tons of questions about different numbers, and the theme is always recurring. Many take notice of the numbers as coinciding with a major shift (in psyche), and my story is no different. I state "wanting to take place" because, as I shared earlier, I have received many inquiries about numbers, 11 11, in particular, and I have witnessed people tap into this and take life to the next level. I have also seen many others miss the clues and or not truly keep the faith and tap all the way in. Without a doubt, 1111 is the most commonly reported number seen. 11 is a portal into an opening, a higher consciousness which is a higher dimension. This is your portal to 4d/5d.

1111

11:11 is the portal, the opening, as previously mentioned. Take a look at the number 1111; it even looks like a portal. This is why it is always seen or noticed at the beginning of the awakening steps. This also explains why the person has no clue or knowledge as to what this frequent occurrence means, but it is here for a reason and it's calling you to lead you to a higher purpose and existence.

My story was no different. I started to see 11:11 as I dug deeper into my livet and spirituality. Everything was still fairly new to me in the holistic world, and I had no clue why I saw this number so much, but I took notice of the regular occurrence. I would begin to tell friends and family, whom probably just thought I was losing my mind. I started to research the number 11:11 and other numbers that are known as angel or master numbers. I found that there was an abundance of others who experienced this divine phenomenon. 11:11 acts as a gate because you are about to enter into a higher portal of consciousness, a new beginning, the one. The number one symbolizes things are coming together in your life. Now, fast forward – you continue to progress, and the number briefly goes away. As you enter the portal, new numbers will occur such as 222, 33, and 44 and so on. This is the time when I really started to ascend. Thus, I had to share this newfound knowledge and growth with others. I would teach and preach the sermon of plant-based livet and spirituality and, a bit later, some friends would ask me about the numbers, saying that the same was happening to them.

I had planted seeds that were starting to sprout.

This is why you have to water and nurture those seeds.

Looking back, I can affirm how important that is, as I gave everyone the same tools to ascend from the 11:11 portal, but only some followed through and achieved this goal. Again, this is why it is so important to tap into those clues at the moment that they are given, especially the moment you see these numbers. The master number may hold the intent of what you desire and want to manifest.

Keep the thoughts positive and pure, and attempt to tap into whatever clues life and the ascended angels may be giving you via your thoughts at the moments; if your thought was not pure, transmute it instantly.

22-33-44-55

Let me preface by saying that none of these master numbers have absolute meaning; they are more or less guides and clues, so one must truly tap into thyself and search for their truth in the meaning. They are signs, not absolute definitions. You have to be attentive to yourself and your personal truth.

From 11:11, if you tap in and tune in, you may move to 22, which is building upon the awakening then acquiring new knowledge and downloads. 33, for me, took on a life of its own. 33 became my life path number which can be a number you may be attached to for the rest of your life. This is extremely helpful, as these are constant reminders and guides, thus angels. The number 33 aligns with master teaching and being guided by ascended master teachers. 33 is a magical number for many reasons and grows occult as the 33 degrees of Freemasonry. There are also 33 vertebrate in the spine which is our life force, our Kundalini.

So, 1111 is a spiritual awakening.

The portal, 22, builds upon the awakening by seeking new knowledge or downloads.

33 has to do with master teaching, healing, and helping enlighten others.

44 is building upon your teaching and knowledge and now manifesting your dreams.

55, then, has to with a major change ahead.

Once again, these are not absolute, and you may see these in conjunction with other numbers. For example, 11:33, or you may not see some at all. For me, I did see 1111 upon awakening. Numbers may progress in succession. This is dependent upon your vortex or flow.

Meditation

From here, it is time to start digging deep and tapping in. You are on the right path and have made room for new downloads to take place. Use your tools again, such as meditation, which will help you tap into the seat of your soul (your third eye.) There are many different ways to meditate.

Let's review the most basic methods. The main keys to meditation for beginners are to have the back straight and eyes closed. Keeping your back straight allows for Kundalini energy, your 33 divine energy to flow from the root chakra, the base of your spine, all the way up the spine and out through your crown chakra, radiating light to the universe. Allowing your eyes to close gently allows you to help your mind come to a rest, not allowing the mind to wander. If your eyes are having trouble coming to a close, you can gently focus on one spot in front of you. This is a powerful visualization meditation. Keep in mind – during meditation, you should not need any crutches like music or a special setting. While these factors may help beginners, the ultimate goal of meditation should be to have the ability to meditate at any time or place, such as while washing dishes, in the shower, or while walking or driving. Being in the now, focusing on what's at hand, is a form of meditation.

We can use deep breathing techniques to help calm us, lower our heart rate, and ease the mind and thoughts. Inhale for a mental count of three, expanding belly, chest not moving, hold inhale for a mental count of three, and exhale for a mental count of three. Come back to this technique at anytime to calm thoughts. If disharmonious thoughts occur during meditation, a powerful tool you can use is to visualize capturing your disharmonious thought in a balloon, holding it on a string, and letting it go. Visualize that you are watching that thought float away. Another tool to use as a form of meditation, or in conjunction with traditional meditation practices, is chanting a mantra which frees the mind.

Chanting different mantras, particularly *Hare Krishna*, can put you in an instant meditative state. Chanting *Hare Krishna* is like a direct number to call on the divine, higher power, source, God, or whatever you like to call it. Hare Krishna is the personal cell number.

Hare Krishna

Hare Krishna

Krishna

Krishna

Hare

Hare

Hare Rama

Hare Rama

Rama

Rama

Hare

Hare

Hare Krishna and *Hare Rama* translate to God. Like the ancient harmonic tone of Om, these words have special spiritual sound vibration. Om is said to be the God frequency; when chanted, it connects you with the divine. Om vibrates at 432 hertz which is the same frequency as everything in nature. A good duration for meditation is 20 minutes or more. Brain scans show drastic brain wave activity calmed at around 20 minutes. However, a few moments are better than none, so start at five to ten minutes, if you have to, and work up to 20 minutes.

Meditation has endless benefits, similar to almost everything else under the wholistic sun. I will share some of the key benefits like increased energy through moments of stillness, calming of thoughts and mind, enhanced clarity, improved focus, reduction of anger and stress, reduction of cortisol, and a tremendous increase in awareness, consciousness, and spirituality as well as the opening of your third eye (your seat to your soul), thus increasing your intuition!

Chakras

Through meditation and awareness of energy and that of others, you can unplug and balance your chakras through addressing and releasing past traumas or current emotional or physical dependencies like vanity, ego, lust, or fear. Technically, there are more than seven energy systems (chakras) within the human body, but let's review the main seven, starting with the root chakra.

The root chakra is located at the base of the spine where the spine and hip connect, and its color is red. Your root chakra is your fundamental base and what you look to for grounding and survival. Fear and such can affect your root chakra. Grounding, earthing, meditation, and an attitude of gratitude can help heal root chakra.

Next, moving upward, is your sacral chakra, located at your hips. This is your reproduction and sexual energy center. This chakra also has to do with creativity and creation. Its color is orange. It can be blocked by past hurt or trauma from previous relationships, guilt, abuse, and low libido. It can be healed through identifying sexual blockages and being aware of past, current, and future partners.

Next, moving up, is your solar plexus chakra which deals with your energy (inner-g) and willpower. Its color is yellow. It can be blocked by ego, lack of emotional control, or shame. It can be healed through balancing emotions and need for control.

Next, moving upward, is your heart chakra, having to do with love, which can be blocked by hate and negativity. The heart chakra is the color green and is located at your heart's center. It can be healed through having more compassion, more love, and service to others.

Next up is your throat chakra, bearing the color blue, deals with your expression or lack thereof. Truth, sat nam, and verbal expression, can be blocked by lack of expression and lies. Can be healed through expressing your truth, articulating your feelings, and even choosing silence at times.

Next is your third-eye chakra, located at the area in between and just above your eyebrows. Your third-eye chakra holds the color energy indigo and has to do with intuition and wisdom. It can be blocked and become calcified from fluoride, babylon tricks, the matrix, illusions and diet. It can be healed by removing fluoride use, chaga mushroom, distilled water, vegan livet, meditation, sun gazing and applied knowledge.

The seventh chakra is your crown chakra, bearing the color purple and having to do with divinity and spiritual connections. It can be blocked by vanity, attachments, lack of knowledge of cellf. It can be healed through cellf exploration, service to others, and workin on lower chakras.

The chakras can be summed up in "I am" form, starting at the root: I am, sacral; I feel, solar plexus; I do, heart; I love, throat; I speak, third eye; I see, and crown; I am divine.

Being unaware of your energy centers cause your energy centers to be open and exposed, thus letting in unwanted energy vampires. This is the main purpose for balancing and healing your chakras. Look at your chakras like a flowing river. If one section of the river is blocked upstream, it will affect the flow of the whole stream. The same goes for your chakras. If one is blocked, it can lead to imbalances in the whole chakra energy (inner-G) system

Meditation also leads you to develop more faith and understanding through the healing, balancing, and aligning of your chakras, also building your intuition and spirituality while opening your third eye.

Yoga/Third Eye

Another powerful tool that you have at your disposal is yoga. Yoga is meditation in motion. Yoga, like much of holistic health, has multiple benefits. Yoga helps tremendously to become more in tune with your body, physically and mentality, helping you in the healing and balancing of your chakras. With flexibility, improved strength, and muscle tone, you will find yourself reaping more benefits.

Becoming in tune with one's body has great benefits. You hold and store stress in your shoulders and back, which manifests in the form of back pain, stiffness, aching, and inflammation. Through yoga, you can target, address, heal, and release those blockages. Originally, yoga was a preparation for sitting in lotus position for extended period of times in meditation. Meditation and yoga allow your Kundalini to rise to your third-eye chakra which is the seat to your soul.

The Third Eye

The third eye, or what is technically referred to as the pineal gland, is the size of a pea and located at the center of your brain next to the pituitary gland. This is the most important gland in your body, as it regulates all of the other glands. The pineal gland regulates and outputs serotonin and melatonin. Serotonin is the feel-good chemical in your body; too little of serotonin equates to depression and mood swings. Melatonin is what relaxes and sends signals to your body to sleep and affects your mood through hormones, neurotransmitters, and circadian rhythm or sleep cycle. Your glands and neurotransmitters are disrupted from the array of daily toxins and chemicals. The third eye, in particular, becomes calcified from the byproduct, fluoride. Thus, most pineal glands are not working at full capacity.

Decalcification of the Third Eye

The first step to decalcifying your pineal gland is to cut out all intake of fluoride via water, mainly. Toothpaste is also the second largest culprit. Fluoride-free toothpaste is a priority as well as a clean, non-tap water source. The pineal gland is like a magnet to fluoride and is deposited into the pineal gland more than any other part of the body, including your bones.

The other key, of course, is one's livet, or lack thereof (diet). Your livet helps detoxify the body and fluoride, just the same. Chaga is one of the greatest tools used to decalcify the pineal gland due to its high antioxidant content. Chaga also has one of the highest antioxidant levels of any food source on Earth, light years away from pomegranate which is generally in second place. What is most important, as related to the third eye, is that chaga contains the highest concentration of melanin that has ever been discovered in any food source. Chaga's favorite food to feed off of, so to speak, is melanin. The third eye produces melatonin, the deep sleep regulator;

however, if the pineal gland is not fed, it cannot work properly, thus not producing enough melatonin that you are unable to get proper, restorative rest. Chaga is the number one source of nutrients for the pineal gland; however, there is no magic solution, so a holistic approach to detoxification must be taken. In conjunction with chaga, you can use items such as green juice with cilantro to detox. Meditation and chanting may also assist in detoxification. Chanting can vibrate and stimulate the pineal gland which will help it secrete beneficial properties. Chanting *Om*, which carries what is said to be the God frequency and the original sound of creation, can directly vibrate and stimulate the pineal gland. Chant with powerful intent, meaning, and feeling.

Lastly, sun gazing can help stimulate and decalcify the pineal gland. You must use caution, though, as you can cause damage to the eyes. The best time to sun gaze is a few seconds before sunrise and sunset. Decalcifying your pineal gland will inevitably open up many new realities and dimensions.

Sacred Geometry and Earthing

The world around you, or rather how you see the world around you, will start to change. You will also become more in tune with the biorhythms of Earth through the stimulation of the pineal gland, thus becoming more in tune with circadian rhythm. You will start to notice things around you in nature like sacred geometry; before that, you will be more encouraged to go outside in nature. You may even feel the urge to want or need to out into nature, barefoot, which is referred to as earthing or grounding. Earthing allows your body to connect with the energy and resonance of the Earth. This should be done barefoot to grass for best effect. While in nature, possibly barefoot, with your green juice, tapped in to source, third eye beaming, you may notice the world will unlock and open up for you. You may start to notice sacred geometry in just about all things in nature from the spider web to the dandelion and sunflower to the pine cones to purple cabbage to Romanesco and so on. The world is built and based on energy, vibration, thoughts, numbers, and sacred geometry. Once you realize and unlock these keys, the world is yours.

Spiritual Warfare

The powers that be, the elite, do not want you to have these keys. They are worried because they know how divinely powerful every person is and that you are born that way. They know that you are an all-powerful co-creator, and they do not want you to have control over your creativity and reality. They wage spiritual and physical warfare upon you through chemicals, frequencies, and silent weapons such as Wi-Fi, 5G, cell towers, cell phones, radio frequency, 440 hertz, smart meters, harp, microwaves, and so on. These can program and harm you by affecting your neurons, not allowing you to critically think and question official narratives. These are silent weapons. 5G is referred to by those with their third eye open as the beast system, the total takeover and control of everything. They are planning to unleash 300,000 Gwen towers, which basically replicate maximum microwave exposure on every corner, all for the sake of social media to run faster?

We think not.

This is about total control over your physical treatment and spiritual health. Keep in mind, the deployment of the 300,000 new towers is the same amount deployed over the last three decades. One must realize and stay conscious of this so one can proactively live a holistic lifestyle and detoxify, daily, because the heavy metals act as an antenna in your body to the frequencies from cell towers. Detoxify, daily, and meditate, daily, to remain level headed and clear. One must be conscious of what goes into the mainframe.

Turn off your cell phone or put in airplane mode during the night while sleeping. You should also unplug Wi-Fi during your sleep cycle. The goal is to limit exposure as you are being bombarded with an array of harmful chemicals and frequencies. This is also why the elite ban items that are beneficial to one's spirituality such as cannabis and psilocybin. Cell phones, laptops, and radiation also lower sperm count, and there are experiments where seeds and plants have been placed next to a Wi-Fi router, proving they will not grow properly, if at all.

Cannabis and Psilocybin

Cannabis and psilocybin have been around long before INI. Cannabis and psilocybin date back to ancient times, making appearances in hieroglyphics, both coming from Mother Earth. Prohibition is less than 100 years old, starting in the 1930's, while the cannabis plant is hundreds of years old. Psilocybin has proven medicinal studies that show it is helpful in treating depression and many are left with the most spiritual experiences they ever had. Johns Hopkins studied the results of 36 adults, showing that one-third reported psilocybin as the single most influential spiritual experience of their life while 80% reported a loss in depression and an overall increase in well-being (Griffiths, 2016). Studies show that brain scans of those under psilocybin influence have similar scans to those in meditative states, showing an overall calming of brain activity. Psilocybin is, in fact, one of the best remedies for depression. Micro-dosages of psilocybin have little to no psychoactive effects yet profound effects on mood, depression, and creativity. You will not be talking to Bart Simpson on this dosage. You likely will not notice psychoactive effects of the dosage at all.

Cannabis has a significant relationship with your body and physiology than you may realize, if you realized this at all. Your body produces THC through its cannabinoid system. That's right, your cannabinoid systems. Did you know your body had such a system? It is also one of the largest and most important systems in your body. The endocannabinoid system is made up of cannabinoid receptors that help the brain and body communicate with nerve cells, maintaining the balance of factors such as sleep, pain, and mood. This is often referred to as the master system. The plant has many broad-spectrum benefits, medicinally, therapeutically, and regarding psychoactivity.

Through the use of cannabis, you can also go into a deeper meditative state. Cannabis and psilocybin, however, should not be used as a crutch. There should be an intention placed prior, that of a deeper meditative state, intentions of expanding, or intentions of healing depression with psilocybin, but not needing to have this to achieve a meditative state. You should not need to use cannabis before meditation, but if you do use it prior, use with intentions to enhance meditation.

Cannabis can be used in many ways; however, when you put fire to it, you must keep in mind and be honest with INI (yourself) that there is little to no medicinal benefits after that. You certainly never want to use blunt and tobacco products that cause cancer and keep you chemically confused and addicted. Healthier alternatives would be to use a quality vaporizer like the volcano. Vaping not only excludes most carcinogens but also releases a further spectrum of medicine. Do not fool yourself to believe that any form of inhalation is healthy for the lungs. So, if you want a healthier alternative from there, consuming via ingesting would be most beneficial. This is where the true medicine exists, in the cannabis oil, which goes by different names such as Rick Simpson Oil (RSO), Full Extract Oil (FECO), or Phoenix Tears.

There are plenty of testimonials available to review including those of children relieved of seizures within seconds with CBD. I will leave you to make your own decisions, as this book is not intended to lend any medical advice, and these statements have not been approved by the FDA (luckily).

Whatever method or modes you choose, be very mindful that many to most growers grow with intentions of profits over patients. So, they often use spray and artificially regulate the growth of the plant through the use of synthetic pesticides and growth enhancers often combined with undetectable mold to the common eye, but are commonly detected with test samples. Growing your own would be the best option if you cannot find a trusted source.

In sum, if you pull forth from your tool belt, you will start to ascend to higher dimensions of reality. This concept of living in different dimensions may seem far out to most, possibly assuming this equates to time travel. That is not the case. You can travel through time when you use your imagination and think of the future or past. Alternate dimensions are alternate perceptions of reality and different levels of consciousness. The concept is that simple, really. 3D is fear-, monetary-, and material-based, and self-serving, while 4d is transmutational dimension leading to 5d which is just the opposite reality, one based on love, eternal riches, and service to others.

Transition to higher dimensions. Ascension can be achieved by cleaning the current, negative matrix programming through your livet, meditation, and thought control, making way for the new programming of our desire.

Choose love, peace, harmony, and health.

Love is Always the Answer

Love, the highest vibration, is always the answer. Love is love, and love is my religion. Any religious foundation is based on love. When choosing love, you will win. Choosing the opposite, death via dead food, will give opposite results. Where is the love in factory, farmed, slaughtered animals for food, never mind the nutrition? Where is the love in your day to day thought process? Choosing negative hateful thoughts will also yield us a much different result as well. Where is the love in the music you listen to and the entertainment that goes into your consciousness, subconscious, and physical, or are they all fear, death, and destruction based?

In Sum

If you've made it this far, I salute you. I appreciate you, and you should congratulate yourcellf. If you stay the course and apply the basic guidelines and tips, you will undoubtedly blast off, or, as I like to say, ascend and live the greatest possible version of yourcellf. Simplify the entire process by ingesting and applying only clean, high-vibration food, thoughts and exercises; then, by natural universal law, under the LOA, you, in turn, will be a pure, high-vibrational hueman (human) or huewoman (hu-woman) being. Health is the true measure of wealth. Wealth has little to do with monetary riches but more with health. How healthy are you and your family?

I very much love and appreciate you for reading this.

Much love peace and respect,
Benevolent Blizz

Sources

Beltran-Aguilar ED, et. al. (2010). Prevalence and Severity of Dental Fluorosis in the United States, 1999-2004. Centers for Disease Control. NCHS Data Brief No. 53.

Choi A., et. al. (2012). Developmental Fluoride Neurotoxicity: A Systematic Review and Meta-Analysis. Environmental Health Perspectives. Jul. 20 (2012).

Griffiths R., Johnson M., et. al. (2016). Psilocybin produces substantial and sustained decreases in depression and anxiety in patients with life-threatening cancer: A randomized double-blind study. Dec. 30 (12): 1181-1197.

Hayes, T.B. (2010). Atrazine induces complete feminization and chemical castration in male African clawed frogs (Xenopus laevis). Proceedings of the National Academy of Sciences, 107(10), 4612-4617. dio:10.1073/pnas.0909519107

National Biomonitoring Program (2017, April 07).
Retrieved from
https://www.cdc.gov/biomonitoring/BisphenolA_F
actSheet.html

New Jersey Department of Health Hazardous Substance
Fact Sheet.
Retrieved from
https://nj.gov/health/eoh/rtkweb/documents/fs/16
99.pdf

Zelko, F. (2018). Toxic Treatment: Fluoride's
Transformation from Industrial Waste to Public
Health Miracle. Origins: Current Events in
Historical Perspective. 11(6) (Mar. 2018).

34530437R00078

Made in the USA
Middletown, DE
31 January 2019